C.C MCCUNE

Emily's OCD

Her story of discovery, learning, and hope

This book was professionally typeset on Reedsy.
Find out more at reedsy.com

Contents

1

Introduction

Navigating Life with OCD

In the pages that follow, we embark on an intimate journey through the labyrinth of Obsessive-Compulsive Disorder (OCD) alongside Emily, a resilient soul navigating the intricate tapestry of childhood, and adolescence. This book serves as a compassionate exploration of outward appearances and internal battles, offering a glimpse into the relentless challenges and triumphant moments that shape Emily's journey with OCD.

Unveiling the Veiled Struggle: The Dance of Concealment and Turmoil

At first glance, Emily may seem like any other individual going through life. Yet, beneath the surface lies a silent struggle against the intrusive thoughts, worries, and compulsive rituals of OCD. Each chapter unveils a layer of this intricate dance—a symphony of concealed battles, concealed resilience, and concealed triumphs.

2

The Masked Smile

In the small suburban town of Willow Creek, where white picket fences lined the streets and every lawn seemed perfectly manicured, lived Emily's family. At first glance, they were the epitome of the American dream – a loving family with two children, Emily and her younger brother, Jake. However, behind the veneer of normalcy, a storm brewed within the walls of their home.

Emily, just eleven years old, was a bright and cheerful child – or so it seemed. Her smile, always ready for the outside world, masked a daily struggle that threatened to consume her. Emily was grappling with Obsessive-Compulsive Disorder (OCD), a condition that hijacked her thoughts and dictated her actions in ways unimaginable to those who only saw her external appearance.

The morning routine at the family household was a delicate ballet of rituals. Emily would meticulously arrange her toys in a specific order before leaving for school, her hands lingering over each item to ensure they were just right. She would then face the mirror, counting to a specific number before deeming herself presentable for the world. The act of leaving the house became an intricate dance of checking and rechecking, an exhausting routine to satisfy the relentless demands of her internal thoughts.

Outside the confines of her home, Emily wore a mask – not the tangible kind but an emotional one, carefully crafted to blend seamlessly with societal expectations. At school, she laughed and engaged in conversations with her peers, skillfully diverting attention away from the internal chaos. Her teachers praised her politeness and diligence, unaware of the mental gymnastics that played out behind her expressive eyes.

The discrepancy between Emily's external appearance and internal turmoil was a silent scream for help, but the world remained oblivious. The lunch breaks spent in isolation, avoiding contact with others to prevent contamination fears, went unnoticed. The constant need to touch and retouch objects, the whispered counting under her breath – all hidden beneath the facade of a well-adjusted child.

Even at home, where her family should have been the first to notice the signs, Emily became a master of disguise. She would strategically time her rituals when her parents were occupied, slipping into the bathroom to wash her hands for the umpteenth time or arranging her belongings in a secret, ritualistic order when she thought no one was watching.

Emily's younger brother, Jake, sensed something out of the ordinary. He witnessed the late-night struggles when Emily would tiptoe around the house, compelled to check and recheck the locks on the doors and windows. Yet, the unspoken rule of secrecy bound him too. The family, unknowingly, tiptoed around the elephant in the room, their love for Emily momentarily blinding them to the cries for understanding.

As the days unfolded, Emily's internal battles intensified, mirroring the building conflict within her family. The difference between the external facade and internal turmoil deepened, creating a situation that seemed insurmountable. Soon, the mask began to crack, revealing the raw truth that lay beneath Emily's carefully constructed smile.

3

Cracks in the Mask

The facade Emily wore grew more fragile with each passing day, and the strain of her internal struggles began to manifest in subtle ways that demanded attention. In the heart of her seemingly perfect life, the cracks in her carefully constructed mask started to show.

One afternoon, as sunlight streamed through Emily's bedroom window, she sat at her desk, hunched over her textbooks. Her once-impeccable notes were now marred by doodles and eraser smudges, evidence of the growing chaos within her mind. The outside world perceived Emily as a diligent student, but the truth was that her thoughts were held captive by an incessant loop of doubts, fears, and worries.

The turning point came during a routine visit to the grocery store with her mother. The neatly organized shelves and gleaming aisles became a battlefield for Emily's mind. Each item she touched demanded an intricate ritual, a silent negotiation to stave off the anxiety that threatened to engulf her. Her mother, preoccupied with the shopping list, remained oblivious to the silent struggle playing out beside her.

As Emily's internal turmoil peaked, her mother, sensing something amiss, turned to her with concern etched on her face. The facade cracked, and tears welled up in Emily's eyes. She mumbled something about feeling unwell and rushed outside. It was in that moment of vulnerability that the truth began to surface.

Back at home, Emily's mother gently approached the subject, her concern radiating through the kitchen. Emily, no longer able to bear the weight of her secret, tentatively began to share her struggles. The counting, the handwashing, the paralyzing fears that dictated her every move – it all spilled out, raw and unfiltered. Her mother, shocked and saddened by the revelation, listened intently, realizing the depth of her daughter's silent suffering.

The family dynamics shifted as the truth about Emily's OCD became a shared burden. The once-unseen struggles now occupied the forefront of their collective thoughts. It was a delicate dance of understanding and acceptance, with each family member trying to understand their own emotions. Jake, Emily's younger brother, harbored a mix of guilt for not speaking up sooner and sadness for the battles his sister fought in silence.

The external support network expanded as the family sought professional help. Therapists and psychologists became allies in the family's journey, guiding them through the maze of OCD. Emily's mother, in particular, became a fierce advocate, researching and learning about OCD to better support her daughter. The stigma that once veiled mental health issues began to dissipate within the family, replaced by a shared commitment to navigate the challenges together.

Despite the newfound openness, Emily continued to wear her mask outside the safety of her home. The school remained a place of secrecy, and the familiar rituals persisted, hidden beneath the surface of her daily schedule and interactions. The difference between her external appearance and internal turmoil persisted, but the family's understanding offered a glimmer of hope that someday the two worlds might align.

4

A Glimpse Into the Mind

In the quiet corners of Emily's mind, a symphony of thoughts played continually, a mixed up melody shaping the rhythm of her everyday life. The manifestations of her Obsessive-Compulsive Disorder (OCD) were as intricate as they were subtle, revealing the complex nature of the disorder that silently shaped her world.

Obsessions: The Uninvited Guests

Emily's obsessions were unwelcome guests in her mind. They arrived unannounced, often taking the form of intrusive thoughts that sparked intense anxiety and discomfort. The fear of contamination, a common theme in OCD, lingered in every corner of her consciousness. Whether it was the touch of a doorknob, the feel of a textbook, or the gentle brush of another person's hand, Emily's mind painted these ordinary experiences with feelings of dread.

As she moved through her daily routine, the obsessions morphed into an unending stream of doubts. Did she step on each tile a certain amount of times? Did she wash her hands with a precise ritual? What if she hadn't locked the front door properly? These doubts, seemingly harmless to an outsider, became unwanted worries that required Emily's attention and appeasement.

The more Emily tried to suppress these thoughts, the more they multiplied. It was an attempt to control the uncontrollable. This internal struggle, hidden behind her masked exterior, summed up the essence of her obsessions in OCD.

Compulsions: The Ritualistic Dance

To counter the overwhelming anxiety induced by obsessions, Emily created habits of compulsions – ritualistic behaviors performed in an attempt to calm the distressing thoughts. These compulsions provided temporary relief but fed the cycle of OCD, reinforcing the belief that the rituals were necessary to prevent harm.

Emily's rituals were as varied as her obsessions. Hand washing became a meticulous ceremony, a ritualistic cleansing to rid herself of imagined contaminants. Counting, a common compulsion in OCD, manifested in the number of steps she took, the times she touched an object, or the repetitions of a phrase under her breath.

One particularly poignant manifestation of Emily's compulsions was the need for symmetry and order. Her belongings, meticulously arranged in specific patterns, served as a desperate attempt to impose order on the chaos within her mind. The external world became a canvas for the internal struggle, and the rituals, seemingly nonsensical to an outsider, were the threads that held Emily's fragile sense of control together.

The Cycle of OCD: A Vicious Loop

OCD operates in a cycle of obsessions and compulsions, a loop that tightens its grip on the individual's thoughts and behaviors. Emily, like many others with OCD, found herself trapped in this cycle, where the temporary relief provided by compulsions was inevitably followed by the resurgence of obsessions.

The more Emily succumbed to her compulsions, the more entrenched they became. The rituals, once a source of comfort, transformed into a prison from which escape seemed impossible. The compulsion to perform these rituals became a reflex, an automatic response to the anxiety provoked by obsessions.

Breaking this cycle required a huge shift in perspective and a commitment to confront the discomfort triggered by obsessions without resorting to compulsions. This therapeutic approach, known as Exposure and Response Prevention (ERP), would later become a crucial part of Emily's journey toward recovery.

The Invisible Struggle: Educating About Childhood OCD

Emily's story serves as a window into the often misunderstood world of childhood OCD. Unlike popular misconceptions, OCD is not merely a quirk or a desire for order; it is a clinically recognized mental health disorder with significant impacts on daily functioning.

Childhood OCD affects approximately 1-2% of the population, and early intervention is crucial for better outcomes. Recognizing the signs is the first step toward providing support. It's essential to dispel the myth that OCD is a matter of personal choice or willpower. The brain circuitry of individuals with OCD operates differently, leading to an overactive threat-detection system that triggers intense anxiety.

The impact of OCD extends beyond the individual, affecting family dynamics and relationships with others. Understanding and empathy play pivotal roles in creating a supportive environment for those navigating the challenges of OCD.

5

Family Dynamics and the Ripple Effect

As Emily's family confronted the reality of her Obsessive-Compulsive Disorder (OCD), the ripples of Emily's invisible struggle extended far beyond the confines of her mind. The family dynamics shifted, revealing the profound impact that mental health challenges can have on interpersonal relationships.

Educating the Family: A Shared Understanding

The first step in navigating the complexities of OCD within the family was education. Armed with knowledge about the disorder, the family began to understand that Emily's behaviors were not a mere rebellion or a passing phase. OCD was a neurological condition, and each seemingly irrational compulsion served a purpose in her internal world.

Understanding OCD as a family meant recognizing that Emily's struggles were not a reflection of inadequate parenting or a lack of discipline. Instead, it was an opportunity for collective support and empathy. The family's journey became a collaborative effort to break down the stigma associated with mental health, both within the household and in the broader community.

Supporting Siblings: Jake's Perspective

While Emily's parents navigated the labyrinth of OCD, her younger brother, Jake, wrestled with his role as a supportive sibling. Siblings of individuals with OCD often bear witness to the challenges but may not fully comprehend the complications of the disorder. Jake, like many siblings, went back and forth between feelings of guilt for not understanding sooner and a desire to shield Emily from judgment.

Education played a crucial role in helping Jake understand his sister's struggles. Sibling support groups, a resource often underutilized, became a safe space for Jake to share his experiences and learn from others facing similar challenges.

Parental Concerns and Resilience

For Emily's parents, the journey was fraught with concerns and feelings of helplessness. The initial shock of discovering their daughter's internal battles gave way to a fierce determination to provide the support she needed. Seeking therapy not only for Emily but also for themselves became a vital component of the family's healing process.

Parental involvement in therapy is a crucial aspect of treating childhood OCD. The family learned strategies to reinforce therapeutic interventions at home, creating a consistent and supportive environment. Through family therapy sessions, they discovered the power of open communication and the importance of setting realistic expectations for Emily's progress.

One of the challenges parents face in supporting a child with OCD is finding the delicate balance between accommodating their child's needs and encouraging independence. While it is natural for parents to want to alleviate their child's distress, the therapeutic approach often involves gradually exposing the child to anxiety-provoking situations without providing immediate relief.

The Ripple Effect: Extended Family and Community

The impact of Emily's OCD reached beyond the immediate family, affecting relationships with extended family members and friends. Well-intentioned advice or casual remarks could inadvertently contribute to the stigma surrounding mental health. Educating the extended family and friends became a means of creating a broader support network for Emily.

Therapeutic Journey: A Ray of Hope

The family embarked on Emily's therapeutic journey with a commitment to confront OCD head-on. Cognitive-Behavioral Therapy (CBT), and specifically Exposure and Response Prevention (ERP), emerged as a cornerstone of their approach.

CBT aims to identify and challenge irrational thoughts and behaviors, offering practical tools for managing anxiety. ERP, a sub type of CBT, exposes individuals to the thoughts, images, and situations that trigger anxiety, gradually helping them develop healthier responses.

In Emily's case, ERP involved systematic exposure to situations that triggered her obsessions while refraining from engaging in compulsive rituals. For instance, she faced situations where she might encounter perceived contaminants without immediately washing her hands. The gradual, controlled exposure allowed her to build resilience against the anxiety that typically accompanied these situations.

The Gradual Unmasking:

As Emily and her family immersed themselves in therapy, the gradual unmasking of her true self began. The rituals that once held her captive slowly loosened their grip. The family, once bound by the silent struggle, discovered a newfound strength in unity.

6

School Life: A Journey of Balance and Growth

The Classroom Dilemma:

As Emily settled into her desk, surrounded by the hum of classmates preparing for the day, the classroom became a theater for her internal struggles. The routine of gathering supplies, arranging notebooks, and positioning her chair occupied her attention in a way that seemed normal to outsiders but concealed the meticulous compulsions dictated by her OCD.

The teacher's instructions for group activities or collaborative projects posed a unique challenge. The fear of contamination, a dominant theme in Emily's obsessions, manifested in the reluctance to share materials or engage in activities that involved physical contact. The internal conflict waged a silent war against the desire to conform to the expectations of a typical school day.

Recognizing the tangible impact of OCD on Emily's academic performance, a collaborative effort between her parents and school faculty resulted in the implementation of educational adjustments. These adjustments, including extended test-taking time, flexible assignment deadlines, and a supportive environment during exams, became indispensable components of her academic toolkit.

The Lunchtime Conundrum:

Lunchtime, typically a social playground for school children, posed a unique challenge for Emily. The fear of contamination, a central theme in her OCD, meant navigating the cafeteria landscape with caution. The tactile nature of communal tables and shared utensils became potential sources of distress.

The school, recognizing the need for a safe space, designated a quiet area for Emily to have lunch. This small but significant adjustment allowed her to enjoy a meal without the overwhelming anxiety that accompanied the communal spaces. The importance of such tailored accommodations cannot be overstated in creating an inclusive educational environment.

The Impact on Social Dynamics:

While the school took proactive measures to support Emily, the social dynamics remained a complex tapestry. Friendships in elementary school often hinge on shared activities and spontaneous interactions, areas where OCD can create significant hurdles.

The fear of judgment or misunderstanding led Emily to conceal her struggles from her peers. The mask she wore at school, much like the one in the outside world, became a shield against potential ridicule or isolation. Educating classmates about OCD, while beneficial, did not eliminate the internal fear of being perceived as different.

Coping Strategies for School Life:

As Emily navigated the intricate terrain of school life, coping strategies emerged as essential tools for managing the challenges posed by OCD.

- 1. Establishing a Routine: Creating a structured daily routine provided a sense of predictability, helping Emily manage the uncertainty that often triggered OCD symptoms.
- 2. Utilizing Breaks Effectively: Short breaks between classes allowed moments for relaxation and regaining composure. Incorporating mindfulness techniques during these breaks became part of Emily's coping repertoire.
- 3. Establishing a Safe Space: Identifying a designated safe space within the school environment offered a refuge during moments of heightened anxiety. This space served as a sanctuary where Emily could practice coping strategies and regain a sense of control.
- 4. Promoting Open Communication: Facilitating open communication with teachers and classmates about OCD proved instrumental. Awareness and understanding within the school community contributed to a more supportive atmosphere.

The Role of Teachers and Peers:

The involvement of teachers and peers played a significant role in shaping Emily's experience of school life with OCD. The awareness and empathy of educators created an environment where she felt understood and accommodated.

Teachers, armed with knowledge about OCD, became allies in fostering a supportive educational journey. Their role extended beyond the traditional boundaries of imparting academic knowledge to actively contributing to Emily's mental health support system.

Peers, when educated about OCD, exhibited compassion and understanding. Friendships that transcended the barriers of stigma became sources of solace for Emily. The importance of peer relationships in mitigating feelings of isolation and fostering acceptance cannot be overstated.

Evolution of Coping Mechanisms:

As Emily progressed through her school years, her coping mechanisms evolved in tandem with her understanding of OCD. The rituals that once consumed significant portions of her day gradually gave way to more adaptive strategies.

Therapeutic interventions, including Cognitive-Behavioral Therapy (CBT) and Exposure and Response Prevention (ERP), played a crucial role in this evolution. The skills acquired in therapy became tools that empowered Emily to navigate school life with increasing autonomy and resilience.The Therapeutic Bridge Between Home and School:

As Emily's therapeutic journey progressed, the bridge between home and school became a crucial focal point. The strategies employed in therapy, particularly Exposure and Response Prevention (ERP), needed to extend beyond the therapeutic setting and integrate seamlessly into the fabric of Emily's daily life.

Gradual Exposure in Educational Settings:

ERP, a cornerstone of Emily's therapeutic journey, involved gradual exposure to anxiety-provoking situations. In the context of school, this meant incrementally facing the challenges that triggered her obsessions and compulsions. The school counselor, in collaboration with Emily's therapist, devised a plan that exposed her to controlled social situations and shared activities.

For instance, group projects, initially a source of anxiety, became opportunities for controlled exposure. The emphasis was not merely on completing the project but on navigating the social aspects without succumbing to compulsions. The support of understanding classmates, educated about Emily's condition, played a pivotal role in this process.

The Role of School Counselors:

School counselors, often unsung heroes in the realm of mental health support, played a crucial role in Emily's journey. Beyond providing emotional support, they became advocates for mental health awareness within the school community. Through workshops, presentations, and accessible resources, they contributed to destigmatizing mental health challenges and fostering an environment of empathy.

Facing Challenges Head-On:

As the school year progressed, so did Emily's ability to face challenges head-on. The once-daunting prospect of group activities or communal spaces transformed into opportunities for growth. The school's commitment to inclusivity and understanding became a testament to the transformative power of education and compassion.

7

Friendships and Isolation

The Mask of Normalcy:

Emily's school days were punctuated by the delicate art of wearing a mask, concealing the intricate rituals that governed her thoughts. Amid the laughter and camaraderie, the mask became both a shield and a barrier. The fear of being labeled as different or facing rejection led Emily to navigate the social landscape with caution.

Friendships, a cornerstone of childhood development, became a terrain fraught with challenges. The rituals that provided a semblance of control in Emily's internal world often clashed with the spontaneity and unpredictability inherent in friendships. The fear of judgment cast a shadow over her interactions, prompting her to meticulously curate the aspects of her life she shared with others.

Friendship Dynamics:

The dynamics of friendships are inherently complex, even without the additional layer of mental health challenges. Childhood friendships often revolve around shared interests, play, and a natural ebb and flow of interactions. For Emily, the fear of contamination and the rituals associated with it introduced a unique set of hurdles.

Common childhood activities, such as playing with shared toys or participating in group games, became potential triggers for Emily's obsessions. The internal dialogue that accompanied these situations created a barrier between her and her peers. The fear of being perceived as odd or unpredictable led her to withdraw from certain social interactions, choosing isolation over the potential judgment of others.

Educating Peers:

One of the pivotal steps in breaking down these barriers was the education of Emily's peers. The school, building on the foundation laid in earlier chapters, organized age-appropriate sessions to familiarize classmates with OCD. These sessions aimed to demystify the condition, fostering understanding and empathy among the children.

Classmates learned that Emily's rituals were not quirks but coping mechanisms. The importance of not making light of or mimicking these behaviors became a part of the school's ethos. These educational efforts were not only instrumental in reducing stigma but also in creating an environment where Emily felt supported and understood.

The Role of Classmates:

Despite the best efforts of educators and school counselors, the responsibility of creating an inclusive environment extended to Emily's classmates. The awareness sessions provided a foundation, but the day-to-day interactions required a continuous commitment to empathy and acceptance.

Classmates played a vital role in extending invitations and finding ways to include Emily in activities without triggering her anxiety. The gradual integration of controlled exposure into group projects or collaborative games allowed Emily to navigate the social landscape with increasing confidence.

The Impact of OCD on Social Development:

OCD's influence on social development is multifaceted, affecting both the individual with the disorder and those in their social circle. For individuals like Emily, the fear of judgment or the anticipation of triggering obsessions can lead to social withdrawal. This isolation, in turn, may contribute to feelings of loneliness and a sense of being misunderstood.

On the flip side, friends and peers may struggle to comprehend the behaviors associated with OCD. The repetitive rituals or avoidance of certain situations may be perceived as peculiar or disruptive. Education, as demonstrated in Emily's school, serves as a bridge, fostering a supportive community that embraces diversity in the face of mental health challenges.

Navigating Friendship Challenges:

As Emily faced the ebbs and flows of friendship dynamics, her therapeutic journey provided tools to navigate the challenges. Cognitive-Behavioral Therapy (CBT), with a focus on Exposure and Response Prevention (ERP), played a crucial role in addressing the fears that fueled her social anxiety.

Exposure exercises gradually introduced Emily to social situations that triggered her obsessions. Whether it was participating in group activities or sharing materials with classmates, each step was a deliberate move toward breaking the cycle of avoidance and anxiety.

Friendship as a Therapeutic Tool:

Recognizing the potential therapeutic value of friendships, Emily's therapist incorporated elements of social interactions into her sessions. Role-playing scenarios or discussing specific social challenges allowed Emily to apply the coping strategies learned in therapy to real-life situations.

The therapeutic focus expanded beyond symptom reduction to building resilience and fostering a positive self-image. Emily, once hesitant to engage in social activities, began to view friendships as opportunities for growth rather than potential sources of anxiety.

The Intersection of OCD and Puberty:

As Emily navigated the challenges of friendships, another layer emerged with the onset of puberty. The hormonal changes associated with adolescence can influence the severity of OCD symptoms. Heightened self-awareness, coupled with societal pressures, can exacerbate the internal struggles faced by individuals like Emily.

The transition to adolescence underscores the importance of ongoing therapeutic support and a holistic approach that addresses not only the specific symptoms of OCD but also the broader challenges associated with growing up.

Building Resilience Through Friendship:

Despite the hurdles, Emily's journey illuminated the resilience that can blossom within the context of understanding friendships. As her classmates embraced her quirks and supported her in facing challenges,

Emily discovered that true friendships could be a source of strength rather than anxiety.

Friendships, once viewed through the lens of potential judgment, became a canvas for self-expression. The understanding cultivated in her social circle allowed Emily to gradually shed the mask of normalcy, revealing her authentic self to those who truly mattered.

Family Support: The Backbone of Resilience:

While friendships became a significant source of support, the backbone of Emily's resilience remained her family. The open communication and collaborative approach established at the beginning of her journey continued to be a bedrock of support. Family therapy sessions provided a forum to discuss the evolving challenges of friendships and social interactions.

8

Adolescence and Self-Identity

As the pages turned in Emily's story, the onset of adolescence brought with it a new chapter, one marked by the intricate dance of self-discovery and the evolving landscape of Obsessive-Compulsive Disorder (OCD). The teenage years, already a tumultuous period of self-identity and growth, posed unique challenges for Emily as she grappled with the complexities of both her internal world and the external expectations of adolescence.

The Adolescent Journey:

Adolescence, often described as a time of storm and stress, encompasses a myriad of physical, emotional, and social changes. For Emily, the hormonal shifts and the increasing awareness of self brought forth a new set of challenges in managing her OCD. The intrusive thoughts that had once been mere whispers became amplified in the echo chamber of adolescent introspection.

The quest for self-identity, a hallmark of adolescence, interwoven with the persistent threads of OCD. The desire to fit in and be perceived as 'normal' clashed with the compulsions that set Emily apart. The fear of judgment intensified, mirroring the amplified emotions inherent in the adolescent experience.

Impact on Self-Identity:

OCD's influence on self-identity during adolescence is profound. The disorder can shape the lens through which individuals perceive themselves and the world around them. For Emily, the compulsions that once provided a semblance of control began to chip away at her self-esteem.

The internal dialogue, fueled by obsessive thoughts, whispered doubts about her worthiness and normalcy. The desire for acceptance warred with the compulsion to conform to rituals, creating a paradox that defined the landscape of her self-identity.

The Impact of OCD on Academic Pressures:

As Emily progressed through her teenage years, the academic pressures inherent in adolescence converged with the challenges posed by OCD. The increasing demands for academic achievement, coupled with the fear of making mistakes, heightened the internal anxiety that fueled her obsessive thoughts.

Educational accommodations, established in earlier years, continued to be crucial in managing the academic impact of OCD. Extended test-taking time, flexibility in assignment deadlines, and a supportive environment for exams became integral components of Emily's academic toolkit.

Parental Support in Adolescence:

The role of Emily's parents evolved as she navigated adolescence. The delicate balance between providing support and fostering independence became a focal point. Parental involvement in therapy sessions remained crucial, offering insights into the evolving challenges Emily faced.

The Role of Medication:

In some cases, the complexities of adolescence may lead to a consideration of medication as part of the treatment plan. Selective serotonin reuptake inhibitors (SSRIs), commonly used in treating OCD, may be prescribed to alleviate symptoms. The decision to introduce medication is often made in consultation with a mental health professional, considering the individual's specific circumstances.

The Road to Self-Discovery:

As Emily traversed the landscape of adolescence, the journey became a process of self-discovery. The therapeutic interventions, social support, and coping strategies paved the way for her to unravel the layers of her identity beyond the confines of OCD. The teenage years, while marked by internal and external challenges, also held the promise of growth and resilience. Emily's journey underscored the transformative power of understanding, acceptance, and the unwavering strength of the human spirit.

9

Hope and the Future

As Emily's journey unfolded, each chapter was woven with threads of resilience, growth, and the transformative power of seeking help. The culmination of her narrative brings us to a chapter of hope and the future—a chapter that extends beyond the shadows of mental health challenges to illuminate the possibilities of a life well-lived. In exploring hope and the future, we delve into the lessons learned, the enduring strength of the human spirit, and the potential for a future where mental health is prioritized and destigmatized.

Reflections on the Journey:

As Emily reflects on the path traveled from childhood to adulthood, the mosaic of experiences comes into focus. The challenges of Obsessive-Compulsive Disorder (OCD) were not merely obstacles but stepping stones that shaped her resilience. The therapeutic interventions, family support, and the decision to seek help collectively crafted a narrative that defied the limitations of mental health challenges.

The journey, although difficult at times, became a source of empowerment. Emily's story is a testament to the idea that hope is not merely wishful thinking but a tangible force cultivated through courage, self-awareness, and the commitment to well-being.

Lessons Learned:

Emily's journey imparts valuable lessons that resonate beyond the realm of mental health challenges. The power of empathy, the importance of open communication, and the transformative nature of seeking help emerge as enduring lessons.

The Strength of Resilience:

Resilience, cultivated through the peaks and valleys of Emily's journey, emerges as a guiding force. The ability to navigate challenges, adapt to transitions, and maintain a sense of agency in the face of OCD's influence reflects the profound strength of the human spirit.

Resilience is not the absence of struggle but the capacity to bounce back from adversity. Emily's story becomes a beacon for others, illustrating that the human spirit possesses an inherent resilience that can weather storms, emerge stronger, and embrace the possibilities that lie ahead.

A Vision for the Future:

The future, as Emily envisions it, extends beyond the confines of mental health challenges. It is a future where individuals feel empowered to seek help without fear of judgment, where support networks are fortified, and where societal attitudes toward mental health are marked by understanding and acceptance.

In this vision for the future, mental health is prioritized as an integral aspect of overall well-being. Schools, workplaces, and communities foster environments that destigmatize mental health challenges, creating spaces where individuals feel safe to share their experiences and seek support.

The Impact on Mental Health Advocacy:

Emily's journey becomes a catalyst for mental health advocacy. The lessons learned, the transformative power of seeking help, and the strength of resilience collectively contribute to a narrative that challenges societal norms and fosters change.

Hope as a Beacon:

Hope, in the context of mental health, is not a fleeting wish but a guiding force that propels individuals forward. Emily's story serves as a beacon of hope for those navigating similar challenges, illuminating the possibility of a future marked by growth, resilience, and fulfillment. Emily's journey inspires others facing mental health challenges. It showcases that, with support, understanding, and the commitment to seeking help, individuals can transcend the limitations of their conditions and lead meaningful lives. The hope embedded in Emily's narrative becomes a collective call to action. It calls on individuals, communities, and institutions to prioritize mental health advocate for destigmatization, and create environments where seeking help is not only accepted but encouraged. Emily envisions a future where mental health challenges are met with empathy rather than judgment, where individuals feel empowered to seek help early, and where societal perceptions of mental health are reshaped. This vision becomes a driving force for ongoing advocacy efforts. Even in the face of mental health challenges, the horizon is adorned with possibilities.

10

Resources

Obsessive compulsive disorder (OCD) in children and teenagers. (2022, December 31). Raising Children Network. https://raisingchildren.net.au/school-age/health-daily-care/school-age-mental-health-concerns/ocd

Sheldon-Dean, H. (2023, February 23). *Teacher's Guide to OCD.* Child Mind Institute. https://childmind.org/guide/teachers-guide-to-ocd-in-the-classroom/

Sreenivas, S. (2022, May 27). *Childhood ADHD vs. OCD: What to Know.* WebMD. https://www.webmd.com/add-adhd/childhood-adhd/adhd-and-ocd

Turning Point Psychological Services. (2023, October 21). *10 Do's and 5 Don'ts for Parents of Kids with OCD.* OCD & Anxiety Clinic | Turning Point Psychology. https://www.turningpointpsychology.ca/blog/children-with-ocd-guidelines-for-parents#:~:text=Most%20people%20with%20OCD%20

Turning Point Psychological Services. (2023b, October 21). *Acceptance and Commitment Therapy (ACT) for OCD*. OCD & Anxiety Clinic | Turning Point Psychology. https://www.turningpointpsychology.ca/blog/act-for-ocd